GET OUT OF SUGAR JAIL

BY DIANE B. MORRIS

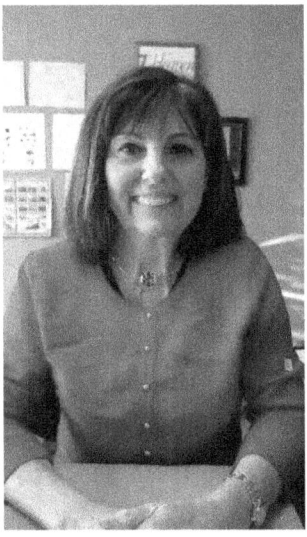

Congratulations on making the commitment to purchase my *Get out of Sugar Jail* book! I am so excited and honored to offer you an easy to implement and permanent solution to smash your sugar cravings in 21 days or less.

My Background:

I am a Registered Licensed Dietitian in the state of Georgia, USA and a Certified Dr. Sear's L.E.A.N. Coach. My passions involve helping individuals take control of their body through proven nutrition practices, mindset and lifestyle adjustments to secure an overall permanent health balance.

My Past:

A wonderful lady lived with our family for over 30 years. She helped take care of my siblings and me while my Mom and Dad worked in their neighborhood grocery store. Every Wednesday, she walked to the bus to go downtown, completed her errands and came home with bags of candies to fill her "magical" candy drawer in her bedroom dresser. The wonderful tasting large German Dark Chocolate bars, Brach's candies and chewing gum were just a few of the candies she carefully placed in this drawer. She often shared these treats with us. So at a very young age, my sweet tooth began to develop. When I was 10 years old, 8 cavities were discovered during one dentist visit! This was one result of my own sugar addiction.

For most of my young adult life, I could eat whatever I wanted and stay a "normal" weight. My body had no trouble metabolizing sugar, or any other foods because my nutrition knowledge helped to keep the pounds off. However, when I hit my forties I gained weight and noticed my waist expanding. My hips were rounder, and it was tough to keep my belly tucked in despite exercising 3 times/week (walking, sit ups, water aerobics, floor exercise programs, etc.).

I experimented with the low fat, high fat, low carb, no carb, and high protein diet rages. I still noticed the nagging belly fat persisting.

At that time, I still didn't realize how sugar and artificial sweeteners caused belly fat, irritability, memory issues and the uncontrollable urges to crave even more sugar!

My Present:

Throughout my 29 years of nutrition practice, medical research and real life experiences, I began to connect the dots and realized that a woman's weight, mood, brain fog, fatigue, gluten sensitivity, and other emotional symptoms are directly related to—uncontrollable real and artificial sugar cravings. I faced them every day myself, now I manage to crush them and keep them under control.

My Future:

I am honored and excited to help individuals finally conquer their struggles with sugar cravings so they can achieve a level of vibrant energy, confidence, joy and get out of their own personal sugar jail.

DISCLAIMER

All information contained within this program is for informational purposes only. It is not intended to diagnose, treat, cure, or prevent any health problem – nor is it intended to replace the advice of a qualified medical practitioner. Always consult your physician or qualified health professional on any matters regarding your health or on any opinions expressed within this program.

What to Expect

In this unique book, I am going to give you everything you need to unlock the key to release you from sugar jail in only 21 days. You can really make this happen, but you can't just read it and expect miracles. You have to implement what you learn and do not quit cold turkey! This program is a gradual transition to eliminate the cravings for good! You will, throughout the process of reading this book, gain your sugar intelligence.

I really truly believe in you and I'm cheering you on to your success!

By the end of this book you will:

1. Be more aware of the impact your sugar cravings have on your thoughts and feelings through a transformational change assessment.

2. Become a master of your sugar intelligence (SI).

3. Detect what a label tells you—Instantly know how much sugar is in a food item to decide whether to put it in your grocery cart or place it back on the shelf.

4. Unlock the 10 keys to eliminate your sugar cravings.

5. Increase your energy and confidence, release the brain fog and experience weight loss.

Note: If your cravings persist, please consult with your doctor to determine if nutrient deficiencies and/or hormones could be the cause. Many people can develop nutrient deficiencies (even when they have a healthy diet). It's common to have hormonal fluctuations and/or imbalances at different stages of our lives. Look for a doctor that specializes in this area.

Section 1: Your Transformational Change

Complete the following assessment to understand your emotions and feelings about your sugar cravings. After 21 days, come back and fill in the blanks to see how far you have come.

I've become aware of the most un-healthy craving(s) I'd like to be freed from:

1.

2.

3.

Three unhealthy feelings and emotions that come from my sugar cravings are (for example, anger, loneliness, depression, sadness, jealousy, resentment):

1.

2.

3.

Three ways these emotions interfere with my life are:

1.

2.

3.

If I was able to overcome this negative pattern on my own, I probably would have conquered them by now, so I am searching help from these 3 resources:

1.

2.

3.

Three good feelings I will enjoy when I eliminate sugar cravings from my body are:

1.

2.

3.

Section 2: Why Do I Have Sugar Cravings?

Cravings are something all of us struggle with at times, so you're not alone if this is something you're dealing with too.

Cravings can be triggered by many things including: sights, sounds, aromas, your environment, stress and more. A perfect example of this is a typical trip to your local mall. Think of walking by the chocolate chip cookie business or cinnamon roll shop – this involves sights, sounds, aromas, AND environment. Another example that is common for a lot of people is stress – stress of a deadline, stress when faced with something you dislike ex: taxes or balancing the check book. Another trigger is boredom.

Since our appetite and our eating habits do not exist in a bubble, experiences that are part of our daily lives can trigger cravings.

The better we understand our cravings, the more equipped we are to deal with them constructively.

It's not realistic to think you will NEVER eat sugar, but the reality is that most people are consuming WAY too much added sugar in their diets. Sugar is in SO many of the foods we eat and we usually aren't even aware of it (bread, crackers, sauces, chips). The worst part of it is, it can be quite addictive.

Your cravings are not always your fault. We are inundated every day with foods that are high in calories and low in nutrients. Fast food, packaged food, junk food, restaurant menus can be very deceiving. Fruit juice may have more sugar than a bottle of Coca Cola! We're ultimately paying the price with our health and our waistlines. When we consume processed foods, nutrient-void foods, our body knows it's not getting what it needs so it craves more and signals us to eat more and more and more. We tend to turn to foods with empty calories that are deficient in necessary nutrients.

Sugar:

The average American consumes about 150 lbs. of sugar per year. That's 12.5 lbs. a month or almost 3 lbs. a week. It's hard to image it's that much! However, you may be thinking, you're not part of the average group because you really don't eat that many sweets. The real problem is that the majority of sugar we consume is hidden in processed and fast foods, cereals, snacks, white flour products - it's even in salad dressings, sauces, and beverages! Even products labeled "healthy" are often loaded with sugar. Gluten free foods tend to have sugar as well.

About 15% of the calories in the American adult diet come from added sugars. That's about 22 teaspoons of added sugar a day! Sugar is usually added to make foods and drinks taste better. Unfortunately, such foods can be high in calories and offer none of the health benefits of fruits and other naturally sweet foods do.

Sugar makes us feel happy, energetic and it can even make us feel calm sometimes.

Here's Why:

The sugar breakdown starts in the mouth and sends signals to the brainstem. From there it goes to another part of the brain that releases dopamine, a neurotransmitter. Dopamine is our "feel good/reward" chemical. This pleasure center is the same center where alcohol, heroin, and cocaine are stimulated. Just when you were feeling "up," you are likely going to feel worse than you did before you had that sugar rush after your blood sugar crashes. So as a result, you want and need even more. It can be a hard cycle to break.

During this immediate sensation, dopamine (a chemical messenger) quickly signals another part of the brain to implant a "memory bank" for future pleasure. Thus, our cravings and addictions continue in a vicious cycle.

Our brain needs a constant fuel (like gas in our car). Gas = glucose. The brain does not have the capacity to store glucose. It is the amount of sugar we consume per day beyond the recommended amount that gets us into sugar jail.

The 2016 American Dietary guidelines recommend we consume less than 10 percent of our daily intake of calories from 'added sugars', as a target to help us meet our nutritional needs, without going over our calorie limit.

Added sugars, sugars added by food manufacturers.

The goal of this book is to follow The American Heart Association guidelines. The AHA recommends a maximum of 6 tsp. of sugar for women (26 grams of sugar) or 100 calories and 9 tsp. for men (37 grams) or 150 calories per day.

There is a great article titled, *Food Cravings Engineered by Industry*, which details how big food companies keep us eating through a combination of science and marketing. Copy this link into your browser to learn more if you're interested:

 http://www.cbc.ca/news/health/food-cravings-engineered-by-industry-1.1395225

Of course there are many possible causes for cravings including but not limited to stress, nutrient deficiencies, hormone imbalances and fluctuations in blood sugar levels. This is another reason why it's good to keep a sugar journal.

A 30-day Sugar and Hydration Daily Journal is included in this book. See sample between Section 2 and 3. I added the journal so that you can become more in tune with what you're craving and what you may be missing in your diet. You may also learn more about the triggers, which are often signals that a change in your diet might be beneficial.

When it comes to sugar in foods and beverages your brain's response is to send the signal to eat more. You might think this is the perfect reason to consume artificially sweetened foods, however, this isn't true.

When you eat a sweet food item that doesn't contain any calories your brain gets confused. This causes you to crave even more sweets.

Sugar in Soda:

Per 12 ounces of soda—Lemon-lime soda contains 37.6 grams of added sugar and ginger ale contains 31.8 grams, each of which is equal to about 9 1/2 teaspoons of sugar. Cola has 38.9 grams of added sugar and pepper-type soda varieties contain 38.2 grams. Cola and pepper-type sodas have about 9 3/4 teaspoons of sugar. Root beer contains 39.2 grams of sugar, which is almost 10 teaspoons of sugar. **Cream soda is among the worst choices** with 49.3 grams per serving or 12 1/3 teaspoons. Grape and orange-flavored sodas contain between 42 and 45 grams of sugar, which is a little more than 10 teaspoons. Keep in mind that if you drink a 16-ounce or 20-ounce bottle of soda, your intake of sugar will be much higher. **Adapted from** Sara Ipatenco, Demand Media healthyeating.sfgate.com

Artificial Sugar Studies:

One study performed MRI's on volunteers while they took sips of water sweetened with sugar or water sweetened with sucralose (Splenda). The scans showed that sugar activates the reward center of the brain while sucralose does not[1].

For this reason, artificially sweetened food and drinks don't fully satisfy cravings for natural sugar in the pleasure/reward center of brain. Ultimately, the artificially sweetened food leaves you craving more.

Sucralose is not the only bad guy. Another study found that Aspartame (Equal) is yet another source for increased cravings and a motivation to eat. Acesulfame K (Sunett, Sweet One), and Saccharin (Sweet'N Low, Necta Sweet) also have the same effect on the brain.

AminoSweet and NutraSweet are two of the newer names for Aspartame.

Finally, because artificial sweeteners are so much sweeter than natural sugar, it confuses up your taste buds. Over time you will require sweeter and sweeter foods and beverages to 'feel like' you are tasting something sweet.

Workbook: Sugar and Hydration Daily Journal

Name: _____ **Day 1** _____

Example (more forms can be found at the end of this book)
- Complete the form by totaling the amount of **water you drink and the sugar grams you consume each day.**
- Use only one form per day. Do not put anything on this form that pertains to another day.
- Record all foods and beverages, including water, you consumed from the time you wake up to the time you go to bed.
- Check the food label to see how many servings the product provides. Example: If there are 2 servings contained in the product, and you consumed the whole package; multiply the sugar grams' x 2.

Food	Portion	Sugar Grams	Water Ounces
TOTAL			

Section 3: Labels

Label Reading Basics:

By learning to read labels, you will be able to find out which foods are good sources of nutrients for your daily intake. The left side of the label shows the **total amounts** of different nutrients **per serving.** The right side shows the % of the daily value for a healthy person (see more about % Daily Value below). When you're reading labels search for low sodium foods, low in saturated fat, no trans-fat, no high fructose corn syrup. Avoid advertisements on the front of the package, as they may be deceiving. Use your sugar intelligence by scanning the Nutrition Facts label.

Nutrition Facts

Per 3/4 cup (175 g)

Amount	% Daily Value
Calories 160	
Fat 2.5 g	4 %
Saturated 1.5 g + Trans 0 g	8 %
Cholesterol 10 mg	
Sodium 75 mg	3 %
Carbohydrate 25 g	8 %
Fibre 0 g	0 %
Sugars 24 g	
Protein 8 g	

Vitamin A	2 %	Vitamin C	0 %
Calcium	17 %	Iron	0 %

Start with The Serving Size

Always read the serving size to ensure this is the amount you will be eating. Look for both the amount for 1 serving size and # of servings in the package. Check your portion size compared to the serving size on the label.

% Daily Value: Gives you a general idea of how a particular food fits into a daily meal plan. This applies to healthy people eating 2,000 calories. Adjust accordingly to your calorie needs, for example, 5% or less is low for all nutrients (you want to limit saturated fat, cholesterol, and sodium). 20% is high (you want to include fiber, calcium, vitamins, and minerals).

Total Fat: Includes the good fats (mono's and poly's), saturated fats, and trans fats.

Sodium: Limit to 1400 – 2400 mg per day.

Protein: Extra lean, organic grass fed, free-range sources are the best choices.

Carbohydrates: Total carbohydrates are comprised of starch (complex carbs), sugar and fiber.

Sugar: Sucrose is table sugar (fructose+glucose), corn sweetener, high-fructose corn syrup, fruit-juice concentrates, nectars, raw sugar, malt syrup, maple syrup, fructose sweeteners, liquid fructose, honey, molasses, anhydrous dextrose. *Words ending in '-ose,' are* chemicals for sugar. If any of these words are among the first few ingredients on a food label, the food is likely high in sugar. The total amount of sugar in a food is listed under 'Total Carbohydrates' on the label.

Referring to the label image above, there are 24 grams of sugar in the product. **There should be less than 2g of sugar for every 5g of carbohydrates.** 1 gram is about the weight of a paper clip.

4 grams = 1 teaspoon

Saturated Fat: Choose foods that contain no more than 2 grams of saturated fat per serving.

Monounsaturated and Polyunsaturated Fats: Are not required on a label. Look for healthy fats such as olive, coconut, flaxseed, and peanut oils.

Trans Fat: Choose foods that do not contain trans fat. 0 grams/day.

Cholesterol: Maximum 300 mg/day.

Fiber: Eat at least 35 grams of fiber/day. This pertains to women as well as men.

Avoid all of these Additives:

- MSG
- Nitrates
- BHT, BHA
- Tartrazine (yellow #5) or other dyes (listed with the name and #)

General Label Reading Rules:

- The first ingredient makes up the largest proportion of a food product and then ingredients are listed in descending order by weight.
- The fewer ingredients, the better.
- If you do not recognize more than 2 ingredients or cannot pronounce them - *DON'T BUY IT.*
- If the words "partially hydrogenated" or "hydrogenated" are in the ingredients list, put the food back. These are hidden trans fats.

Identify the Words Derived from 'Sugar'

Natural Sugars

- ✓ Honey
- ✓ Coconut or palm sugar/sweetener
- ✓ Pure maple syrup
- ✓ Molasses
- ✓ Barley malt syrup
- ✓ Brown rice syrup
- ✓ Fruit puree/concentrate
- ✓ Evaporated cane juice
- ✓ Organic cane sugar
- ✓ Brown sugar
- ✓ Raw sugar
- ✓ Turbinado sugar

Un-Natural Sugars

- ✓ White sugar
- ✓ Corn syrup
- ✓ High-fructose corn syrup
- ✓ Fructose
- ✓ Glucose
- ✓ Sucrose
- ✓ Dextrose
- ✓ Maltodextrin
- ✓ Mannitol
- ✓ Sorbitol
- ✓ Sorghum
- ✓ Xylitol

Sweetness-Artificial and Natural Sugar Substitutes Comparison Table

Know your Sweeteners!

Here is a comparison 'sweetness' list for artificial sugars and natural sugar substitutes.

Artificial Sweetener	Brand Names	Sweetness as compared to Sugar
Aspartame	Equal®, NutraSweet®, others	180 times sweeter than sugar
Acesulfame-K	Sunett®, Sweet One®	200 times sweeter than sugar
Saccharin	Sweet'N Low®, Necta Sweet®, others	300 times sweeter than sugar
Sucralose	Splenda®	600 times sweeter than sugar

Natural Sugar Substitutes: Stevia and Monk Fruit

Stevia:

There are a lot of Stevia products out there on the market that are mixed with other chemicals and artificial sweeteners. Check the label before you buy any. It should say 'Stevia' and nothing else. The FDA approved only the purified form of Stevia, called Stevioside, as safe to use. If you see whole Stevia leaves or crude Stevia extracts at your local natural foods store, don't buy them. Buy the natural sugar substitute called Stevia.

Stevia is about 100 to 300 times sweeter than sugar, but has no carbohydrates, calories, or artificial ingredients. Stevia is natural, unlike other sugar substitutes. It's made from a leaf related to popular yellow garden flowers, like asters and chrysanthemums called Sweetleaf.

Not everyone likes the way it tastes. Some people find it bitter, but others think Stevia tastes like menthol.

Look for a powder or liquid form of Stevia in grocery stores and health-food stores. You can cook with it as well! Each brand has its own Sugar-to-Stevia Ratio, so check the package before you measure out sweeteners.

Monk Fruit:

Monk fruit is a deliciously sweet fruit that can be used as a healthy way to sweeten foods and beverages without all the added calories of sugar. In Asia, monk fruit is a traditional food that has been used for centuries as a low-calorie functional beverage and food ingredient. Monk fruit is grown in orchards, nestled amongst the mountains of Southern China where it has been cultivated for hundreds of years. Monk fruit is GRAS (Generally Recognized as Safe) by the FDA. Monk fruit seedlings and fruit are GMO-free and monk fruit juice and extract contain no artificial chemicals. Monk fruit juice concentrate is a natural fruit juice that is 15-20 times sweeter than sugar. Monk fruit extract is 150-200 times sweeter than sugar and is supplied in a concentrated powder form. This delicious fruit provides natural, low-calorie sweetness from fruit without all the calories of sugar. However, it may not be recommended for a cooking substitute.[3]

Be A Label Detective: Making Sense of Product Terms (Label Reading)

Keyword	What they mean
Free	An amount so small, health experts consider it nutritionally insignificant.
Sodium free	Less than 5 mg sodium*.
Cholesterol free	Less than 2 mg cholesterol, and low in saturated fat (includes a restriction on trans fat)*. Not necessarily low in total fat.
Low	Always associated with a very small amount.
Low fat	3 G or less fat*.
Low in saturated fat	2 G or less of saturated and trans fat combined*.
Reduced	At least 25% less of a nutrient compared with a similar product.
Reduced in Calories	At least 25% less energy than the food to which it is being compared.
Source	Always associated with a significant amount.
Source of fiber	2 Grams or more fiber*.
Good source of calcium	165 Mg or more of calcium*.
Light	When referring to the nutritional characteristic of a product, this can only appear on foods that are either "reduced in fat" or "reduced in energy" (calories) explanation on the label of what makes the food "light"; this is also true if "light" refers to sensory characteristics, such as "light in colour"**.

*Per reference amount and per serving of stated size (specific amount of food listed in "Nutrition Facts")

**Three exceptions that do not require an explanation are "light maple syrup", "light rum" and "lightly salted" with respect to fish. Note that a separate provision is made for the claim, "lightly salted", which may be used when a food contains at least 50% less added sodium compared with a similar product.

Section 5: 12 Keys to Get Out of Sugar Jail

Here are the 12 keys for your road to success. Unlock your mind, body and spirit to a whole new world of getting out of sugar jail! I am excited you have utilized all the tools in this book in your 21-day journey. These 12 keys will give your taste buds a chance to adjust without too much of a shock as you **reduce sugar consumption gradually. This is not a cold turkey process!**

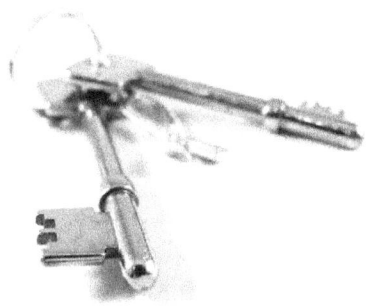

Key#1. Make a Decision: Make a conscious decision to get a handle on your cravings and know that you will conquer them. Cravings most frequently only last 5 minutes. If true hunger is calling your name, you will have hunger pangs. If it is your brain talking to you, it is not a true hunger. Stay grounded and centered. Grab a drink of water with lemon, take a quick walk, call a friend, meditate, take 10 deep breaths, listen to music, dance, say 10 'gratitude's' out loud. Believe me, the yearning for the 'sugar high' will eventually subside.

Key#2. Get White Out of Sight: Crackers, pasta, potatoes, white bread, except cauliflower are refined sugars, which are quickly digested and absorbed as the simple sugar, glucose. Reduce the amount of sugar in recipes. Many times, you can substitute unsweetened applesauce in place of sugar. Cinnamon, nutmeg or apple pie spice are great solutions to add flavor to desserts.

Key#3. Don't Skip Meals: When we skip meals, we may believe we're reducing our calories for the day. The problem is that by mid-afternoon, hunger hits with a vengeance. We then give in to temptation and get mad at ourselves for failing. This often leads to eating even MORE empty calories, more sugar and more processed food. We again feel we are starving and we're stressed out by our failure.

Space your meals at least 4 hours apart with no snacking. Snacks in the morning and afternoon signal your insulin to go into fat storing mode. When you can spread out your meals as evenly as possible throughout the day, ensure that your meal choice is based on whole foods and as a result your blood sugar is likely to be more stable. Half your plate should be designated for your fruit and vegetable selections. Sugar cravings are our body's response to needing energy. By eating balanced meals throughout the day, our energy levels stay up, thereby reducing cravings. Additionally, finish your evening meal at least 3 hours before bedtime.

Key#4. Avoid Bringing the Cravings Home: If you want to make good choices, only keep good choices in the house. Keep the veggies and fruit at eye level and in plain view for the children to see. When they see healthier choices first, they go for what's within easy reach. Keep washed, pre-cut veggies with a yummy dip ready to eat. Stock your pantry with whole foods with fiber to satisfy your hunger and give your body the best nutrition it needs. This greatly aids to the reduction of cravings, because you won't feel so hungry.

Key#5. Eat Protein and Healthy Fats at Each Meal: The low fat diet craze caused people to fear all sources of dietary fat, including the healthy fats that our bodies need to function properly. Healthy fat is crucial to providing essential fatty acids, the absorption of vital nutrients, vitamins and minerals. They are a source of energizing fuel. To make up for the lack of fat and taste in their products, food companies add more SUGAR! Low fat foods are not very satisfying, which causes even more hunger. This leads to grabbing other foods and more calories, which is not good if your end goal is weight loss.

The more we choose whole foods, the less junk food we crave. Our bodies need real food – whole food in its natural state - to thrive and survive. The body knows what it needs to keep it in balance to reduce addictive cravings. L-glutamine is an amino acid that helps improve your brain functioning. Along with glucose, it's one of the main fuels for your brain cells. It improves your ability to sleep, decreases anxiety and reduces cravings. Fresh, raw spinach and parsley are good sources.

If eliminating junk food from your pantry shelves is a challenge for you because your children or spouse have snacks they 'must have', begin to replace one type of snack at a time. For example: Maybe instead of Doritos or Fritos, which are full of artificial ingredients and MSG, choose organic chips. Have salsa or guacamole in the fridge and serve with a plate of fresh cut veggies. Starting with small changes and transitioning little by little can avoid a major mutiny from loved ones. Make simple changes. This can take some time, but it's good to introduce new foods and see what everyone likes. You never know what may become a new favorite!

Key#6. Mediterranean Meal Plan: The typical "Mediterranean" meal includes higher levels of fish, olive oil, fruits, vegetables, cereals and wine. These food choices have been found to be protective against age-related cognitive decline. This type of diet delivers higher amounts of omega-3 fatty acids (from fish), monounsaturated fatty acids (from olive oil and other vegetables), antioxidants (from fruits, vegetables and wine), and B vitamins (from cereal) than the typical Western diet. All of these foods are beneficial to both heart health and brain health, especially because they avoid the bad saturated fat and excess sugar.

Key#7. The B Vitamins and Antioxidants: Thiamin, niacin, folate, vitamin B6 and vitamin B12 are all crucial for brain health. Adequate levels of thiamin, niacin, vitamin B6 and vitamin B12 are needed for the efficient absorption of glucose, the brain's primary fuel. Folate, vitamin B6 and vitamin B12 are involved in the metabolic cycle that regulates homocysteine, an amino acid formed during the breakdown of protein. Elevated homocysteine has been shown to be a risk factor for impaired cognitive abilities in the elderly related to Alzheimer's disease.

Oxidative damage occurs as a result of biochemical breakdowns that release unstable molecules called 'free radicals'. The free radicals attack cell membranes and other cellular structures. The brain is very rich in fats that are vulnerable to oxidation. Oxidative damage to brain cells is strongly implicated in Alzheimer's disease and other forms of cognitive decline. Choosing more antioxidants in your diet will protect the cells against the free radical invasion. Blueberries, raspberries, cranberries, pomegranates, concord grapes, black currant, blackberries, elderberries, artichokes are examples of foods that have high antioxidant levels.

Key#8. The 'Good Fats': Unsaturated fats, or the 'good fats' promote heart and brain health. These include fish oil, flax oil, olive oil, and nut oils. Choose fish options such as tuna, salmon, herring and monounsaturated fats from plant foods (olive oil and tree nuts). Avoid partially hydrogenated oils such as corn oil, cottonseed oil, palm kernel oil, sunflower oil, safflower oil, and soybean oil. Unsaturated fatty acids are critical components of brain cell membranes and are needed for the production and proper functioning of neurotransmitters, these are the chemical messengers our brain cells use to communicate. The polyunsaturated fatty acid- DHA (docosahexaenoic acid), often called "omega-3," is comprised of up to 50% of total fatty acids in the gray matter of the brain and is believed to exert a major influence on neural composition and function.

Key#9. Exercise: Complement your healthy eating choices with regular physical activity. This will reduce the risk of chronic disease. When combined with healthy eating habits, regular physical activity will help you maintain a healthy weight and avoid those sugar cravings throughout the day and night.

Key#10. Get Restful Sleep: What a person does during the day influences how well you sleep at night. Junk food and junk thoughts during the day can cause interrupted sleep cycles. Feeling tired, stressed and exhausted will trigger food binges. When we're tired, we get stressed more easily. Research, published in the American Journal of Human Biology, explains that short or poor quality sleep is linked to obesity. Our appetite can increase when we're tired. Studies show how signals from the brain, which control appetite regulation, are impacted by decreased sleep. Our body craves more energy and we get more energy from food, so we end up eating more, and usually end up making less healthy choices. The best number of hours of sleep is 7-8.5 hours. **Ghrelin, a hormone, stimulates the appetite. It is released into the blood stream during poor quality and a limited quantity of sleep, thus increasing the chances of craving more sugar.**

Key#11. Avoid Caffeine: Caffeine increases cortisol (stress hormone) and epinephrine, which triggers a faster heart rate, higher blood pressure and stimulates the release of insulin. Insulin levels normally increases after you eat. Insulin stimulates the cells in your liver, muscles and fat tissue to absorb glucose. A study published in the July 2004 issue of "The American Journal of Clinical Nutrition" suggested that caffeine induces a state of insulin resistance in your cells, which prompts your pancreas to produce even more insulin than it typically would in response to a meal. Insulin resistance can be particularly troublesome for diabetics or overweight individuals. Reduce the amount of sugar by a teaspoon or two of what you usually put in.

Key#12. Be a Food Label Detective: We've been taught to look at the calories and fat content on labels, but not the actual INGREDIENTS. It's shocking what our food is made up of these days. When we consume sugar, we CRAVE more sugar so it's important to know where it's lurking. I have provided excellent label reading tools in this program for you to master your sugar intelligence. Words like 'healthy,' 'natural,' 'baked,' 'whole grain', etc. are deceiving. For example, Baked Lays Potato Chips contain more sugar than Regular Lays Potato Chips! You wouldn't even think there would *be* sugar in potato chips.

Congratulations for completing your first steps to conquer your sugar cravings!

Looking to find more keys to your health?

Schedule a

Complimentary

Cravings Breakthrough Session

with me at: dianebmorrisrd@gmail.com

To Your Best Health,

Diane

References

1.Frank GK, Oberndorfer TA, Simmons AN, et al. Sucrose activates human taste pathways differently from artificial sweetener. Neuroimage. 2008;39: 1559-69.

2. Blundell JE, Hill AJ. Paradoxical effects of an intense sweetener (aspartame) on appetite. Lancet. 1986 May 10; 1(8489):1092-3

3. Resource: Monk Fruit.org

Workbook: Sugar and Hydration Daily Journal

Name: _____ **Day 1** _____

- Complete the form by totaling the amount of **water you drink and the sugar grams you consume each day.**
- Use only one form per day. Do not put anything on this form that pertains to another day.
- Record all foods and beverages, including water, you consumed from the time you wake up to the time you go to bed.
- Check the food label to see how many servings the product provides. Example: If there are 2 servings contained in the product, and you consumed the whole package; multiply the sugar grams' x 2.

Food	Portion	Sugar Grams	Water Ounces
TOTAL			

Workbook: Sugar and Hydration Daily Journal

Name: _____ **Day 2** _____

- Complete the form by totaling the amount of **water you drink and the sugar grams you consume each day.**
- Use only one form per day. Do not put anything on this form that pertains to another day.
- Record all foods and beverages, including water, you consumed from the time you wake up to the time you go to bed.
- Check the food label to see how many servings the product provides. Example: If there are 2 servings contained in the product, and you consumed the whole package; multiply the sugar grams' x 2.

Food	Portion	Sugar Grams	Water Ounces
TOTAL			

Workbook: Sugar and Hydration Daily Journal

Name: _____ **Day 3** _____

- Complete the form by totaling the amount of **water you drink and the sugar grams you consume each day.**
- Use only one form per day. Do not put anything on this form that pertains to another day.
- Record all foods and beverages, including water, you consumed from the time you wake up to the time you go to bed.
- Check the food label to see how many servings the product provides. Example: If there are 2 servings contained in the product, and you consumed the whole package; multiply the sugar grams' x 2.

Food	Portion	Sugar Grams	Water Ounces
TOTAL			

Workbook: Sugar and Hydration Daily Journal

Name: _____ **Day 4** _____

- Complete the form by totaling the amount of **water you drink and the sugar grams you consume each day.**
- Use only one form per day. Do not put anything on this form that pertains to another day.
- Record all foods and beverages, including water, you consumed from the time you wake up to the time you go to bed.
- Check the food label to see how many servings the product provides. Example: If there are 2 servings contained in the product, and you consumed the whole package; multiply the sugar grams' x 2.

Food	Portion	Sugar Grams	Water Ounces
TOTAL			

Workbook: Sugar and Hydration Daily Journal

Name: _____ **Day 5** _____

- Complete the form by totaling the amount of **water you drink and the sugar grams you consume each day.**
- Use only one form per day. Do not put anything on this form that pertains to another day.
- Record all foods and beverages, including water, you consumed from the time you wake up to the time you go to bed.
- Check the food label to see how many servings the product provides. Example: If there are 2 servings contained in the product, and you consumed the whole package; multiply the sugar grams' x 2.

Food	Portion	Sugar Grams	Water Ounces
TOTAL			

Workbook: Sugar and Hydration Daily Journal

Name: _____ **Day 6** _____

- Complete the form by totaling the amount of **water you drink and the sugar grams you consume each day.**
- Use only one form per day. Do not put anything on this form that pertains to another day.
- Record all foods and beverages, including water, you consumed from the time you wake up to the time you go to bed.
- Check the food label to see how many servings the product provides. Example: If there are 2 servings contained in the product, and you consumed the whole package; multiply the sugar grams' x 2.

Food	Portion	Sugar Grams	Water Ounces
TOTAL			

Workbook: Sugar and Hydration Daily Journal

Name: _____ **Day 7** _____

- Complete the form by totaling the amount of **water you drink and the sugar grams you consume each day.**
- Use only one form per day. Do not put anything on this form that pertains to another day.
- Record all foods and beverages, including water, you consumed from the time you wake up to the time you go to bed.
- Check the food label to see how many servings the product provides. Example: If there are 2 servings contained in the product, and you consumed the whole package; multiply the sugar grams' x 2.

Food	Portion	Sugar Grams	Water Ounces
TOTAL			

Workbook: Sugar and Hydration Daily Journal

Name: _____ **Day 8** _____

- Complete the form by totaling the amount of **water you drink and the sugar grams you consume each day.**
- Use only one form per day. Do not put anything on this form that pertains to another day.
- Record all foods and beverages, including water, you consumed from the time you wake up to the time you go to bed.
- Check the food label to see how many servings the product provides. Example: If there are 2 servings contained in the product, and you consumed the whole package; multiply the sugar grams' x 2.

Food	Portion	Sugar Grams	Water Ounces
TOTAL			

Workbook: Sugar and Hydration Daily Journal

Name: _____ **Day 9** _____

- Complete the form by totaling the amount of **water you drink and the sugar grams you consume each day.**
- Use only one form per day. Do not put anything on this form that pertains to another day.
- Record all foods and beverages, including water, you consumed from the time you wake up to the time you go to bed.
- Check the food label to see how many servings the product provides. Example: If there are 2 servings contained in the product, and you consumed the whole package; multiply the sugar grams' x 2.

Food	Portion	Sugar Grams	Water Ounces
TOTAL			

Workbook: Sugar and Hydration Daily Journal

Name: _____ **Day 10** _____

- Complete the form by totaling the amount of **water you drink and the sugar grams you consume each day.**
- Use only one form per day. Do not put anything on this form that pertains to another day.
- Record all foods and beverages, including water, you consumed from the time you wake up to the time you go to bed.
- Check the food label to see how many servings the product provides. Example: If there are 2 servings contained in the product, and you consumed the whole package; multiply the sugar grams' x 2.

Food	Portion	Sugar Grams	Water Ounces
TOTAL			

Workbook: Sugar and Hydration Daily Journal

Name: _____ **Day 11** _____

- Complete the form by totaling the amount of **water you drink and the sugar grams you consume each day.**
- Use only one form per day. Do not put anything on this form that pertains to another day.
- Record all foods and beverages, including water, you consumed from the time you wake up to the time you go to bed.
- Check the food label to see how many servings the product provides. Example: If there are 2 servings contained in the product, and you consumed the whole package; multiply the sugar grams' x 2.

Food	Portion	Sugar Grams	Water Ounces
TOTAL			

Workbook: Sugar and Hydration Daily Journal

Name: _____ **Day 12** _____

- Complete the form by totaling the amount of **water you drink and the sugar grams you consume each day.**
- Use only one form per day. Do not put anything on this form that pertains to another day.
- Record all foods and beverages, including water, you consumed from the time you wake up to the time you go to bed.
- Check the food label to see how many servings the product provides. Example: If there are 2 servings contained in the product, and you consumed the whole package; multiply the sugar grams' x 2.

Food	Portion	Sugar Grams	Water Ounces
TOTAL			

Workbook: Sugar and Hydration Daily Journal

Name: _____ **Day 13** _____

- Complete the form by totaling the amount of **water you drink and the sugar grams you consume each day.**
- Use only one form per day. Do not put anything on this form that pertains to another day.
- Record all foods and beverages, including water, you consumed from the time you wake up to the time you go to bed.
- Check the food label to see how many servings the product provides. Example: If there are 2 servings contained in the product, and you consumed the whole package; multiply the sugar grams' x 2.

Food	Portion	Sugar Grams	Water Ounces
TOTAL			

Workbook: Sugar and Hydration Daily Journal

Name: _____**Day 14** _____

- Complete the form by totaling the amount of **water you drink and the sugar grams you consume each day.**
- Use only one form per day. Do not put anything on this form that pertains to another day.
- Record all foods and beverages, including water, you consumed from the time you wake up to the time you go to bed.
- Check the food label to see how many servings the product provides. Example: If there are 2 servings contained in the product, and you consumed the whole package; multiply the sugar grams' x 2.

Food	Portion	Sugar Grams	Water Ounces
TOTAL			

Workbook: Sugar and Hydration Daily Journal

Name: _____ **Day 15** _____

- Complete the form by totaling the amount of **water you drink and the sugar grams you consume each day.**
- Use only one form per day. Do not put anything on this form that pertains to another day.
- Record all foods and beverages, including water, you consumed from the time you wake up to the time you go to bed.
- Check the food label to see how many servings the product provides. Example: If there are 2 servings contained in the product, and you consumed the whole package; multiply the sugar grams' x 2.

Food	Portion	Sugar Grams	Water Ounces
TOTAL			

Workbook: Sugar and Hydration Daily Journal

Name: _____**Day 16** _____

- Complete the form by totaling the amount of **water you drink and the sugar grams you consume each day.**
- Use only one form per day. Do not put anything on this form that pertains to another day.
- Record all foods and beverages, including water, you consumed from the time you wake up to the time you go to bed.
- Check the food label to see how many servings the product provides. Example: If there are 2 servings contained in the product, and you consumed the whole package; multiply the sugar grams' x 2.

Food	Portion	Sugar Grams	Water Ounces
TOTAL			

Workbook: Sugar and Hydration Daily Journal

Name: _____**Day 17** _____

- Complete the form by totaling the amount of **water you drink and the sugar grams you consume each day.**
- Use only one form per day. Do not put anything on this form that pertains to another day.
- Record all foods and beverages, including water, you consumed from the time you wake up to the time you go to bed.
- Check the food label to see how many servings the product provides. Example: If there are 2 servings contained in the product, and you consumed the whole package; multiply the sugar grams' x 2.

Food	Portion	Sugar Grams	Water Ounces
TOTAL			

Workbook: Sugar and Hydration Daily Journal

Name: _____ **Day 18** _____

- Complete the form by totaling the amount of **water you drink and the sugar grams you consume each day.**
- Use only one form per day. Do not put anything on this form that pertains to another day.
- Record all foods and beverages, including water, you consumed from the time you wake up to the time you go to bed.
- Check the food label to see how many servings the product provides. Example: If there are 2 servings contained in the product, and you consumed the whole package; multiply the sugar grams' x 2.

Food	Portion	Sugar Grams	Water Ounces
TOTAL			

Workbook: Sugar and Hydration Daily Journal

Name: _____**Day 19** _____

- Complete the form by totaling the amount of **water you drink and the sugar grams you consume each day.**
- Use only one form per day. Do not put anything on this form that pertains to another day.
- Record all foods and beverages, including water, you consumed from the time you wake up to the time you go to bed.
- Check the food label to see how many servings the product provides. Example: If there are 2 servings contained in the product, and you consumed the whole package; multiply the sugar grams' x 2.

Food	Portion	Sugar Grams	Water Ounces
TOTAL			

Workbook: Sugar and Hydration Daily Journal

Name: _____ **Day 20** _____

- Complete the form by totaling the amount of **water you drink and the sugar grams you consume each day.**
- Use only one form per day. Do not put anything on this form that pertains to another day.
- Record all foods and beverages, including water, you consumed from the time you wake up to the time you go to bed.
- Check the food label to see how many servings the product provides. Example: If there are 2 servings contained in the product, and you consumed the whole package; multiply the sugar grams' x 2.

Food	Portion	Sugar Grams	Water Ounces
TOTAL			

Workbook: Sugar and Hydration Daily Journal

Name: _____ **Day 21** _____

- Complete the form by totaling the amount of **water you drink and the sugar grams you consume each day.**
- Use only one form per day. Do not put anything on this form that pertains to another day.
- Record all foods and beverages, including water, you consumed from the time you wake up to the time you go to bed.
- Check the food label to see how many servings the product provides. Example: If there are 2 servings contained in the product, and you consumed the whole package; multiply the sugar grams' x 2.

Food	Portion	Sugar Grams	Water Ounces
TOTAL			

Workbook: Sugar and Hydration Daily Journal

Name: _____ **Day 22** _____

- Complete the form by totaling the amount of **water you drink and the sugar grams you consume each day.**
- Use only one form per day. Do not put anything on this form that pertains to another day.
- Record all foods and beverages, including water, you consumed from the time you wake up to the time you go to bed.
- Check the food label to see how many servings the product provides. Example: If there are 2 servings contained in the product, and you consumed the whole package; multiply the sugar grams' x 2.

Food	Portion	Sugar Grams	Water Ounces
TOTAL			

Workbook: Sugar and Hydration Daily Journal

Name: _____ **Day 23** _____

- Complete the form by totaling the amount of **water you drink and the sugar grams you consume each day.**
- Use only one form per day. Do not put anything on this form that pertains to another day.
- Record all foods and beverages, including water, you consumed from the time you wake up to the time you go to bed.
- Check the food label to see how many servings the product provides. Example: If there are 2 servings contained in the product, and you consumed the whole package; multiply the sugar grams' x 2.

Food	Portion	Sugar Grams	Water Ounces
TOTAL			

Workbook: Sugar and Hydration Daily Journal

Name: _____**Day 24** _____

- Complete the form by totaling the amount of **water you drink and the sugar grams you consume each day.**
- Use only one form per day. Do not put anything on this form that pertains to another day.
- Record all foods and beverages, including water, you consumed from the time you wake up to the time you go to bed.
- Check the food label to see how many servings the product provides. Example: If there are 2 servings contained in the product, and you consumed the whole package; multiply the sugar grams' x 2.

Food	Portion	Sugar Grams	Water Ounces
TOTAL			

Workbook: Sugar and Hydration Daily Journal

Name: _____**Day 25** _____

- Complete the form by totaling the amount of **water you drink and the sugar grams you consume each day.**
- Use only one form per day. Do not put anything on this form that pertains to another day.
- Record all foods and beverages, including water, you consumed from the time you wake up to the time you go to bed.
- Check the food label to see how many servings the product provides. Example: If there are 2 servings contained in the product, and you consumed the whole package; multiply the sugar grams' x 2.

Food	Portion	Sugar Grams	Water Ounces
TOTAL			

Workbook: Sugar and Hydration Daily Journal

Name: _____ **Day 26** _____

- Complete the form by totaling the amount of **water you drink and the sugar grams you consume each day.**
- Use only one form per day. Do not put anything on this form that pertains to another day.
- Record all foods and beverages, including water, you consumed from the time you wake up to the time you go to bed.
- Check the food label to see how many servings the product provides. Example: If there are 2 servings contained in the product, and you consumed the whole package; multiply the sugar grams' x 2.

Food	Portion	Sugar Grams	Water Ounces
TOTAL			

Workbook: Sugar and Hydration Daily Journal

Name: _____**Day 27** _____

- Complete the form by totaling the amount of **water you drink and the sugar grams you consume each day.**
- Use only one form per day. Do not put anything on this form that pertains to another day.
- Record all foods and beverages, including water, you consumed from the time you wake up to the time you go to bed.
- Check the food label to see how many servings the product provides. Example: If there are 2 servings contained in the product, and you consumed the whole package; multiply the sugar grams' x 2.

Food	Portion	Sugar Grams	Water Ounces
TOTAL			

Workbook: Sugar and Hydration Daily Journal

Name: _____ **Day 28** _____

- Complete the form by totaling the amount of **water you drink and the sugar grams you consume each day.**
- Use only one form per day. Do not put anything on this form that pertains to another day.
- Record all foods and beverages, including water, you consumed from the time you wake up to the time you go to bed.
- Check the food label to see how many servings the product provides. Example: If there are 2 servings contained in the product, and you consumed the whole package; multiply the sugar grams' x 2.

Food	Portion	Sugar Grams	Water Ounces
TOTAL			

Workbook: Sugar and Hydration Daily Journal

Name: _____ **Day 29** _____

- Complete the form by totaling the amount of **water you drink and the sugar grams you consume each day.**
- Use only one form per day. Do not put anything on this form that pertains to another day.
- Record all foods and beverages, including water, you consumed from the time you wake up to the time you go to bed.
- Check the food label to see how many servings the product provides. Example: If there are 2 servings contained in the product, and you consumed the whole package; multiply the sugar grams' x 2.

Food	Portion	Sugar Grams	Water Ounces
TOTAL			

Workbook: Sugar and Hydration Daily Journal

Name: _____ **Day 30** _____

- Complete the form by totaling the amount of **water you drink and the sugar grams you consume each day.**
- Use only one form per day. Do not put anything on this form that pertains to another day.
- Record all foods and beverages, including water, you consumed from the time you wake up to the time you go to bed.
- Check the food label to see how many servings the product provides. Example: If there are 2 servings contained in the product, and you consumed the whole package; multiply the sugar grams' x 2.

Food	Portion	Sugar Grams	Water Ounces
TOTAL			

Workbook: Sugar and Hydration Daily Journal

Name: _____ **Day 31** _____

- Complete the form by totaling the amount of **water you drink and the sugar grams you consume each day.**
- Use only one form per day. Do not put anything on this form that pertains to another day.
- Record all foods and beverages, including water, you consumed from the time you wake up to the time you go to bed.
- Check the food label to see how many servings the product provides. Example: If there are 2 servings contained in the product, and you consumed the whole package; multiply the sugar grams' x 2.

Food	Portion	Sugar Grams	Water Ounces
TOTAL